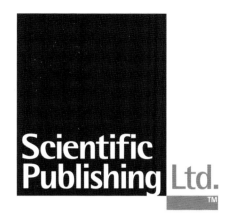

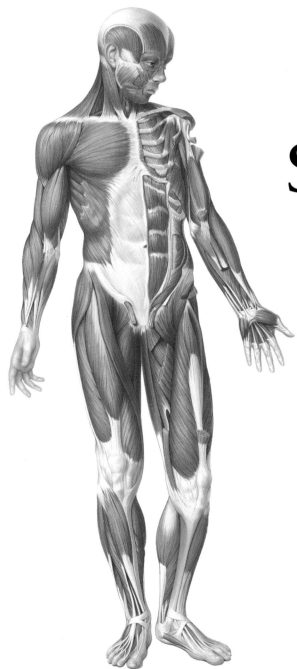

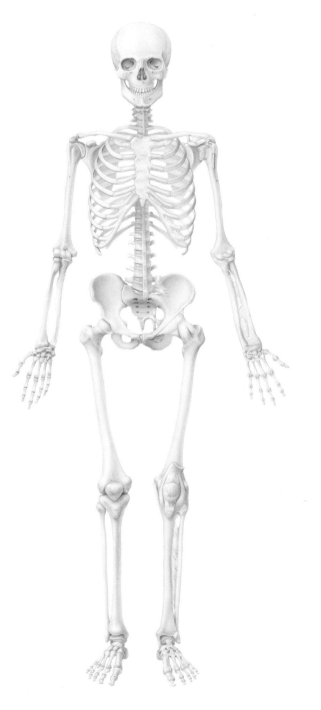

SYSTEMS

of the

HUMAN BODY

An introductory overview of the anatomical systems of the human body

Scientific Publishing Ltd.
www.scientificpublishing.com

Table of Contents

WORKSHEETS: *6 – 8.5" x 11" reproducible anatomical study guides*

- *The Skeletal System: Ossicles*
- *The Nervous System: Brain*
- *The Vascular System: Heart*
- *The Respiratory System: Breathing*
- *The Lymphatic System: Lymph Node*
- *The Digestive System: Overview*

ISBN: 978-1-935612-23-0 Item# HBSF

Published in the United States by: Scientific Publishing Ltd. 167 Joey Drive, Elk Grove Village, IL 60007
Printed in China

The Integumentary System / Skin

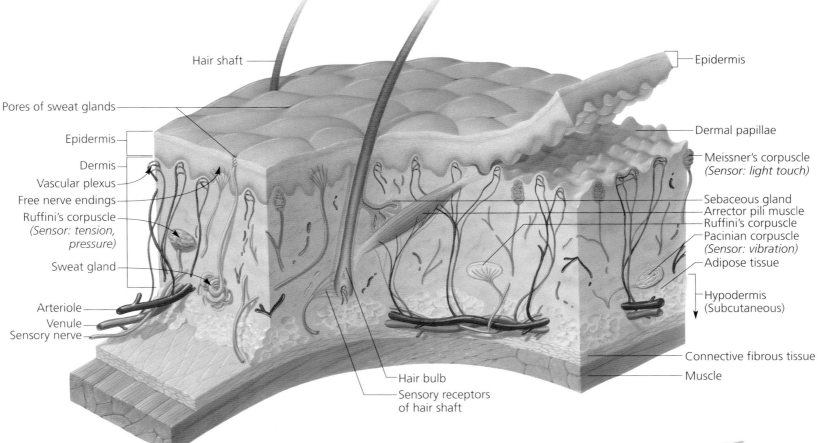

- Hair shaft
- Pores of sweat glands
- Epidermis
- Dermis
- Vascular plexus
- Free nerve endings
- Ruffini's corpuscle *(Sensor: tension, pressure)*
- Sweat gland
- Arteriole
- Venule
- Sensory nerve
- Epidermis
- Dermal papillae
- Meissner's corpuscle *(Sensor: light touch)*
- Sebaceous gland
- Arrector pili muscle
- Ruffini's corpuscle
- Pacinian corpuscle *(Sensor: vibration)*
- Adipose tissue
- Hypodermis (Subcutaneous)
- Connective fibrous tissue
- Muscle
- Hair bulb
- Sensory receptors of hair shaft

Inside the skin

The skin is a highly elastic organ covering the entire outer surface of the body. It performs numerous functions essential to survival, including:

- Prevention of fluid loss from body tissues
- Regulation of normal body temperature
- Maintenance of calcium levels
- Reception of heat, cold, and pain sensations
- Protection against environmental toxins and microorganisms

The three basic layers within the skin are the epidermis, dermis, and subcutaneous layers.

Epidermis
The thin uppermost layer consists of basal cells, melanocytes (responsible for skin color), keratin-producing cells (for hair, nails, and outer protective skin surfaces), Langerhans cells (important in immune protection), and Merkel cells (involved in sensation).

Dermis
The dense middle layer contains the skin's structural components: nerves, blood vessels, sweat glands, hair follicles, sebaceous glands, and collagen.

Subcutaneous
The underlying layer of fat cells cushions body tissues from trauma, insulates against cold, and stores fuel reserves.

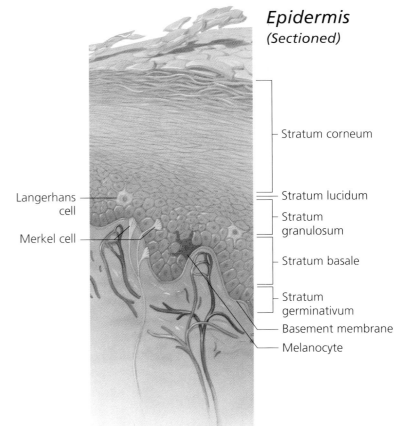

Epidermis
(Sectioned)

- Langerhans cell
- Merkel cell
- Stratum corneum
- Stratum lucidum
- Stratum granulosum
- Stratum basale
- Stratum germinativum
- Basement membrane
- Melanocyte

The Skeletal System

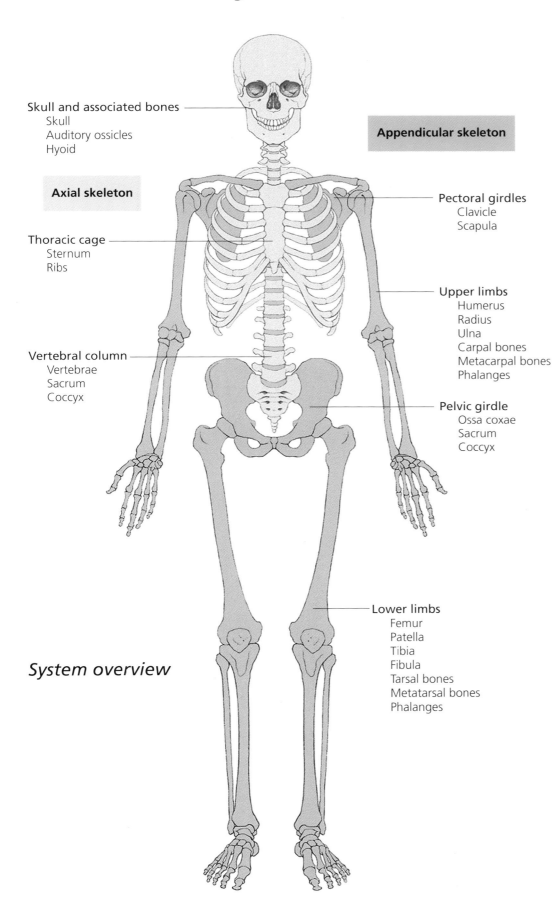

Skull and associated bones
Skull
Auditory ossicles
Hyoid

Axial skeleton

Appendicular skeleton

Thoracic cage
Sternum
Ribs

Vertebral column
Vertebrae
Sacrum
Coccyx

Pectoral girdles
Clavicle
Scapula

Upper limbs
Humerus
Radius
Ulna
Carpal bones
Metacarpal bones
Phalanges

Pelvic girdle
Ossa coxae
Sacrum
Coccyx

Lower limbs
Femur
Patella
Tibia
Fibula
Tarsal bones
Metatarsal bones
Phalanges

System overview

The skeletal system

The skeletal system provides structure and support, forming the framework for the body. The skeleton works together with the muscular system to allow a wide variety of motions, including standing, sitting, and running. In addition to providing support and structure, the skeletal system has several other functions. Bones store minerals, especially calcium, and lipids (in the yellow bone marrow) as reserves. The red bone marrow is the site for blood cell production, including red blood cells, white blood cells, and platelets. The skeletal system is organized into two sections — the axial and the appendicular skeletons, as shown by the system overview diagram.

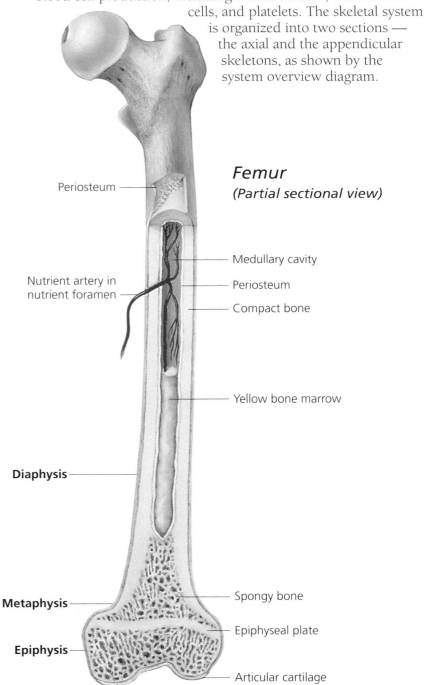

Femur
(Partial sectional view)

Periosteum

Nutrient artery in nutrient foramen

Medullary cavity

Periosteum

Compact bone

Yellow bone marrow

Diaphysis

Metaphysis

Spongy bone

Epiphyseal plate

Epiphysis

Articular cartilage

The Skeletal System

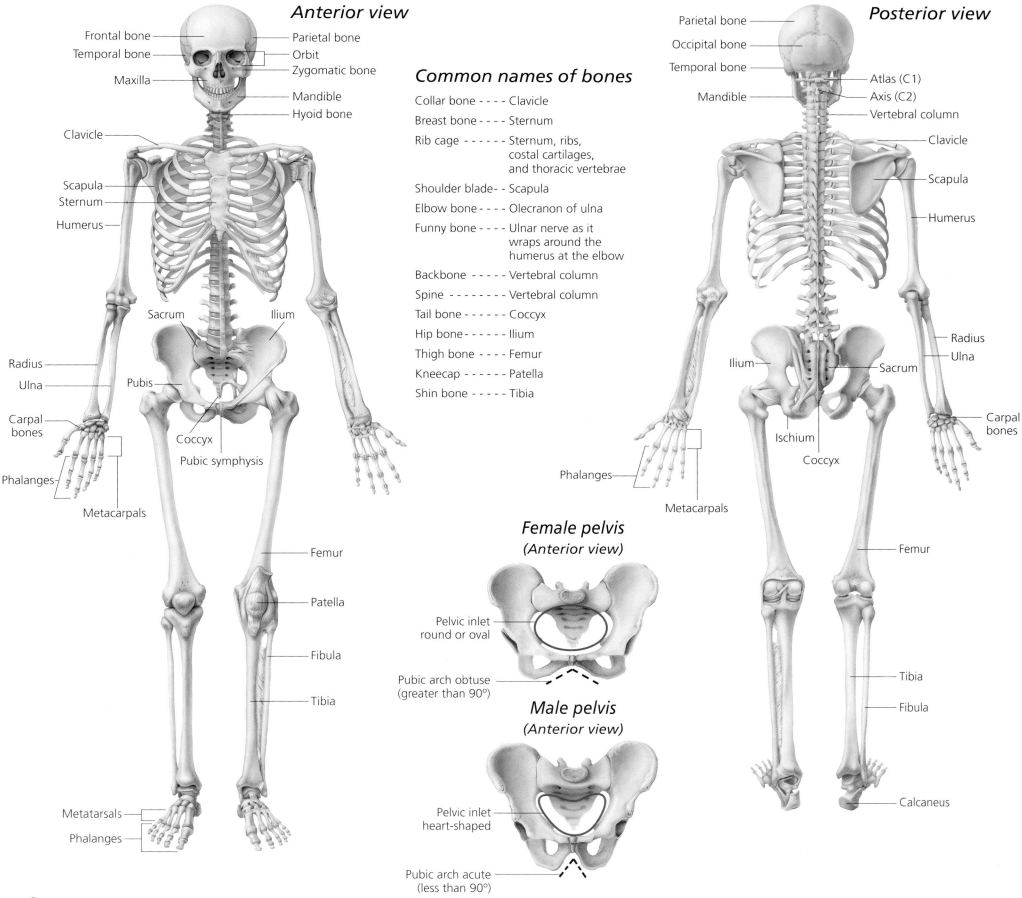

Anterior view

- Frontal bone
- Temporal bone
- Maxilla
- Parietal bone
- Orbit
- Zygomatic bone
- Mandible
- Hyoid bone
- Clavicle
- Scapula
- Sternum
- Humerus
- Sacrum
- Ilium
- Radius
- Ulna
- Pubis
- Carpal bones
- Coccyx
- Pubic symphysis
- Phalanges
- Metacarpals
- Femur
- Patella
- Fibula
- Tibia
- Metatarsals
- Phalanges

Common names of bones

Collar bone - - - - Clavicle
Breast bone - - - - Sternum
Rib cage - - - - - - Sternum, ribs, costal cartilages, and thoracic vertebrae
Shoulder blade - - Scapula
Elbow bone - - - - Olecranon of ulna
Funny bone - - - - Ulnar nerve as it wraps around the humerus at the elbow
Backbone - - - - - Vertebral column
Spine - - - - - - - Vertebral column
Tail bone - - - - - Coccyx
Hip bone - - - - - Ilium
Thigh bone - - - - Femur
Kneecap - - - - - - Patella
Shin bone - - - - - Tibia

Posterior view

- Parietal bone
- Occipital bone
- Temporal bone
- Mandible
- Atlas (C1)
- Axis (C2)
- Vertebral column
- Clavicle
- Scapula
- Humerus
- Ilium
- Sacrum
- Radius
- Ulna
- Ischium
- Coccyx
- Carpal bones
- Phalanges
- Metacarpals
- Femur
- Tibia
- Fibula
- Calcaneus

Female pelvis
(Anterior view)

- Pelvic inlet round or oval
- Pubic arch obtuse (greater than 90°)

Male pelvis
(Anterior view)

- Pelvic inlet heart-shaped
- Pubic arch acute (less than 90°)

The Muscular System

Anterior view

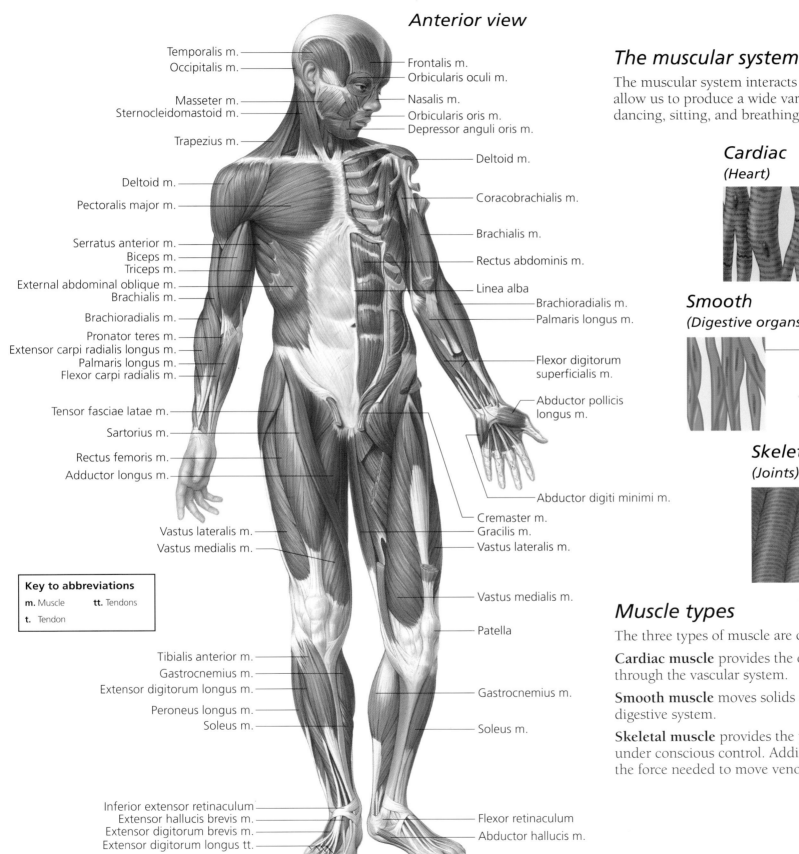

Temporalis m.
Occipitalis m.
Masseter m.
Sternocleidomastoid m.
Trapezius m.
Deltoid m.
Pectoralis major m.
Serratus anterior m.
Biceps m.
Triceps m.
External abdominal oblique m.
Brachialis m.
Brachioradialis m.
Pronator teres m.
Extensor carpi radialis longus m.
Palmaris longus m.
Flexor carpi radialis m.
Tensor fasciae latae m.
Sartorius m.
Rectus femoris m.
Adductor longus m.
Vastus lateralis m.
Vastus medialis m.

Frontalis m.
Orbicularis oculi m.
Nasalis m.
Orbicularis oris m.
Depressor anguli oris m.
Deltoid m.
Coracobrachialis m.
Brachialis m.
Rectus abdominis m.
Linea alba
Brachioradialis m.
Palmaris longus m.
Flexor digitorum superficialis m.
Abductor pollicis longus m.
Abductor digiti minimi m.
Cremaster m.
Gracilis m.
Vastus lateralis m.
Vastus medialis m.
Patella
Gastrocnemius m.
Soleus m.

Tibialis anterior m.
Gastrocnemius m.
Extensor digitorum longus m.
Peroneus longus m.
Soleus m.

Inferior extensor retinaculum
Extensor hallucis brevis m.
Extensor digitorum brevis m.
Extensor digitorum longus tt.

Flexor retinaculum
Abductor hallucis m.

Key to abbreviations

m. Muscle	**tt.** Tendons		
t. Tendon			

The muscular system

The muscular system interacts with the skeletal system to allow us to produce a wide variety of motions, including dancing, sitting, and breathing.

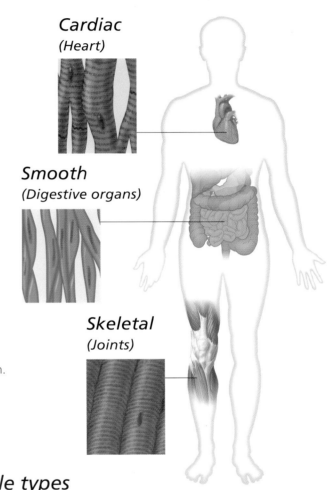

Cardiac
(Heart)

Smooth
(Digestive organs)

Skeletal
(Joints)

Muscle types

The three types of muscle are cardiac, smooth, and skeletal.

Cardiac muscle provides the overall force to move the blood through the vascular system.

Smooth muscle moves solids and fluids through the digestive system.

Skeletal muscle provides the power that enables us to move under conscious control. Additionally, skeletal muscle provides the force needed to move venous blood back to the heart.

The Muscular System

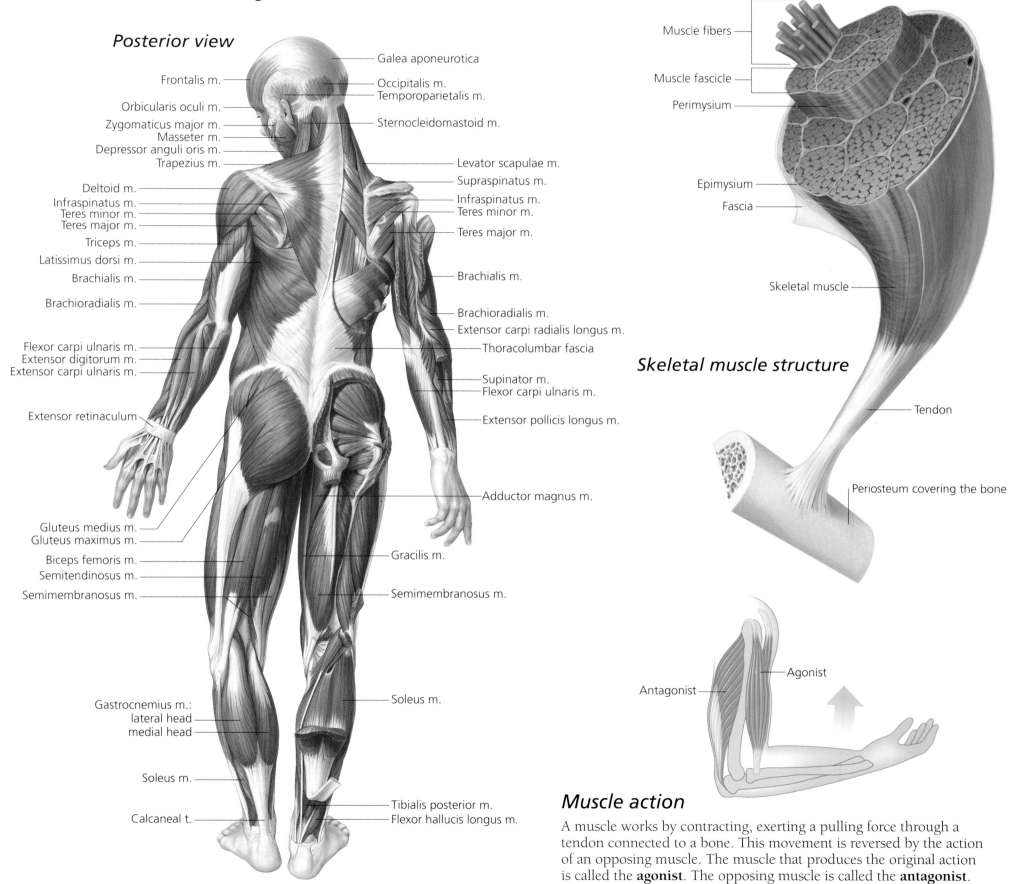

Posterior view

- Frontalis m.
- Orbicularis oculi m.
- Zygomaticus major m.
- Masseter m.
- Depressor anguli oris m.
- Trapezius m.
- Deltoid m.
- Infraspinatus m.
- Teres minor m.
- Teres major m.
- Triceps m.
- Latissimus dorsi m.
- Brachialis m.
- Brachioradialis m.
- Flexor carpi ulnaris m.
- Extensor digitorum m.
- Extensor carpi ulnaris m.
- Extensor retinaculum
- Gluteus medius m.
- Gluteus maximus m.
- Biceps femoris m.
- Semitendinosus m.
- Semimembranosus m.
- Gastrocnemius m.:
  - lateral head
  - medial head
- Soleus m.
- Calcaneal t.

- Galea aponeurotica
- Occipitalis m.
- Temporoparietalis m.
- Sternocleidomastoid m.
- Levator scapulae m.
- Supraspinatus m.
- Infraspinatus m.
- Teres minor m.
- Teres major m.
- Brachialis m.
- Brachioradialis m.
- Extensor carpi radialis longus m.
- Thoracolumbar fascia
- Supinator m.
- Flexor carpi ulnaris m.
- Extensor pollicis longus m.
- Adductor magnus m.
- Gracilis m.
- Semimembranosus m.
- Soleus m.
- Tibialis posterior m.
- Flexor hallucis longus m.

Skeletal muscle structure

- Muscle fibers
- Muscle fascicle
- Perimysium
- Epimysium
- Fascia
- Skeletal muscle
- Tendon
- Periosteum covering the bone

Muscle action

A muscle works by contracting, exerting a pulling force through a tendon connected to a bone. This movement is reversed by the action of an opposing muscle. The muscle that produces the original action is called the **agonist**. The opposing muscle is called the **antagonist**.

- Agonist
- Antagonist

The Nervous System

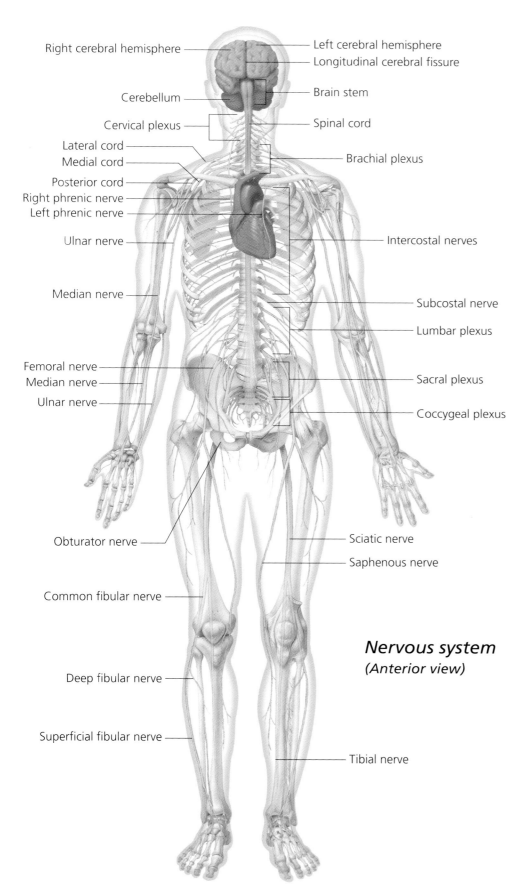

Right cerebral hemisphere
Left cerebral hemisphere
Longitudinal cerebral fissure
Cerebellum
Brain stem
Cervical plexus
Spinal cord
Lateral cord
Medial cord
Brachial plexus
Posterior cord
Right phrenic nerve
Left phrenic nerve
Ulnar nerve
Intercostal nerves
Median nerve
Subcostal nerve
Lumbar plexus
Femoral nerve
Median nerve
Sacral plexus
Ulnar nerve
Coccygeal plexus
Obturator nerve
Sciatic nerve
Saphenous nerve
Common fibular nerve
Deep fibular nerve
Superficial fibular nerve
Tibial nerve

*Nervous system
(Anterior view)*

The nervous system

The nervous system is composed of two integrated subdivisions that are responsible for conducting and processing sensory and motor information: the central nervous system (CNS) and the peripheral nervous system (PNS), which connects the CNS to the rest of the body.

The CNS includes the brain and spinal cord, which are covered by protective membranes called **meninges** (dura mater, arachnoid, and pia mater). The brain processes and coordinates all neural signals received from the spinal cord as well as its own nerves, such as the olfactory and optic nerves. It also performs complex mental functions such as thinking and learning.

Structural division of the nervous system

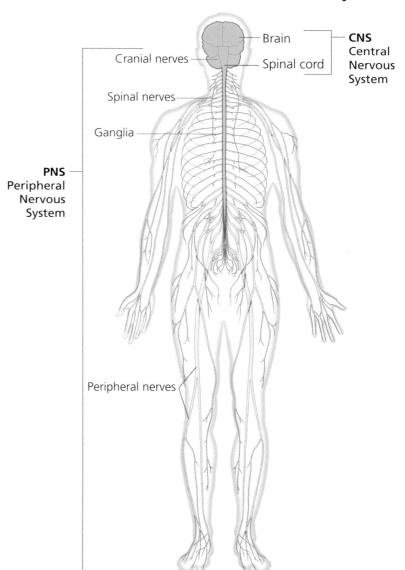

Cranial nerves
Brain
Spinal cord
CNS
Central
Nervous
System
Spinal nerves
Ganglia
PNS
Peripheral
Nervous
System
Peripheral nerves

The Endocrine System

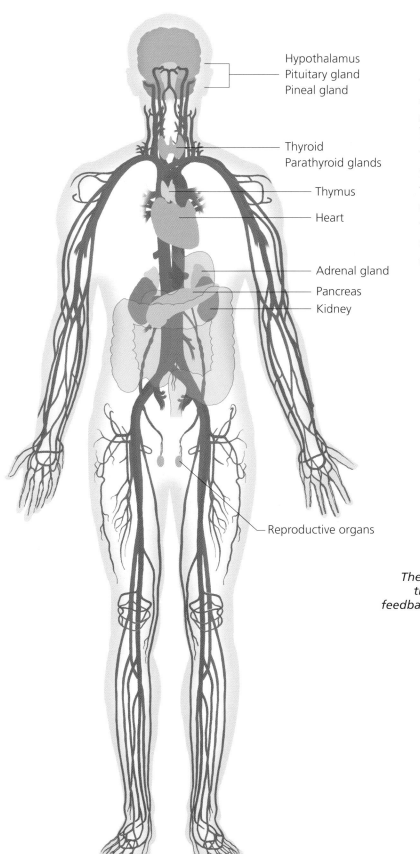

Hypothalamus
Pituitary gland
Pineal gland

Thyroid
Parathyroid glands

Thymus

Heart

Adrenal gland

Pancreas

Kidney

Reproductive organs

The endocrine system

The endocrine system is made up of organs and glands that produce **hormones**, internal chemical messengers that regulate and control functions within the body. Hormones are secreted into the bloodstream and trigger activity within a specific organ or tissue by binding to designated receptors to transmit information.

The endocrine system regulates body processes including metabolism and energy balance, reproduction, growth and development, smooth and cardiac muscle contraction, and blood volumes of substances such as sodium and glucose. The activities of the endocrine system are closely coordinated with the nervous system.

The major organs and glands of the endocrine system include the hypothalamus, thymus, pancreas, ovaries, and testes, as well as the pituitary, pineal, thyroid, adrenal, and parathyroid glands.

The endocrine system and hormones

The release of hormones is controlled by feedback from different parts of the body. Bursts of hormones are released into the blood in response to signals from the nervous system, as well as by changes in blood chemistry and the actions of other hormones. When sufficient levels of a specific hormone reach the target tissue, stimulation of the hormone-producing organ stops and hormone blood levels decrease.

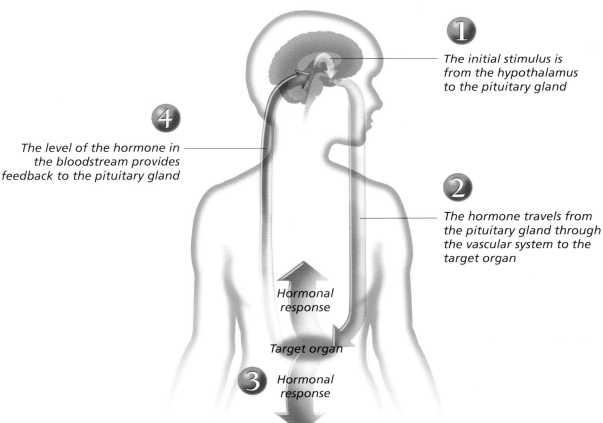

1 *The initial stimulus is from the hypothalamus to the pituitary gland*

4 *The level of the hormone in the bloodstream provides feedback to the pituitary gland*

2 *The hormone travels from the pituitary gland through the vascular system to the target organ*

Hormonal response

Target organ

3 *Hormonal response*

The Vascular System

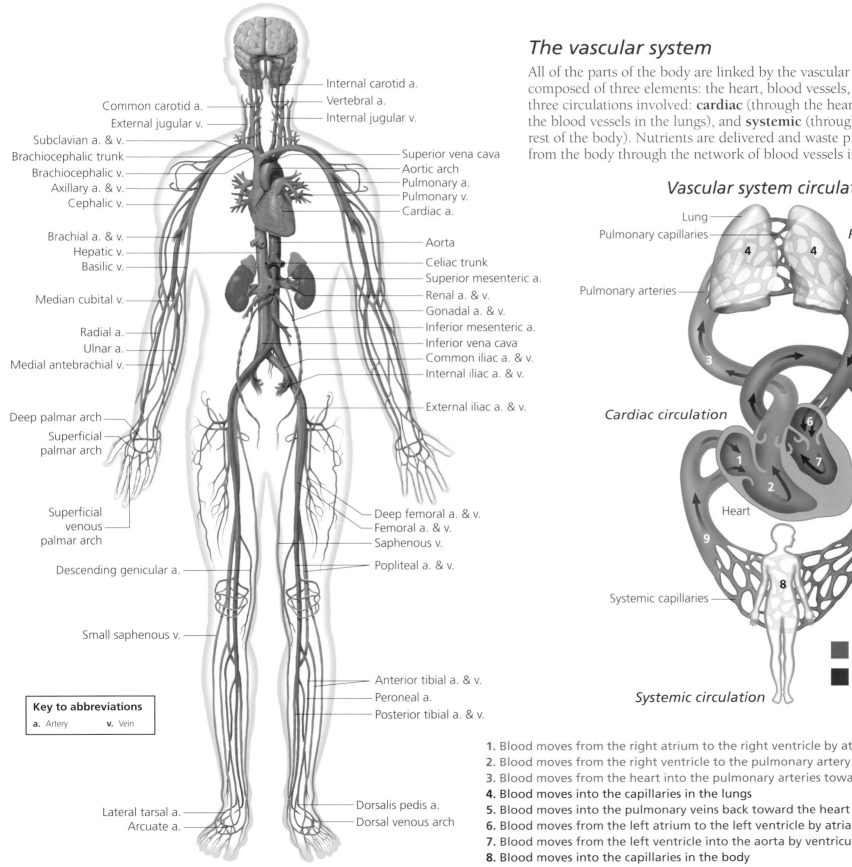

Common carotid a.
External jugular v.
Subclavian a. & v.
Brachiocephalic trunk
Brachiocephalic v.
Axillary a. & v.
Cephalic v.

Brachial a. & v.
Hepatic v.
Basilic v.

Median cubital v.

Radial a.
Ulnar a.
Medial antebrachial v.

Deep palmar arch
Superficial palmar arch

Superficial venous palmar arch

Descending genicular a.

Small saphenous v.

Lateral tarsal a.
Arcuate a.

Internal carotid a.
Vertebral a.
Internal jugular v.

Superior vena cava
Aortic arch
Pulmonary a.
Pulmonary v.
Cardiac a.

Aorta
Celiac trunk
Superior mesenteric a.
Renal a. & v.
Gonadal a. & v.
Inferior mesenteric a.
Inferior vena cava
Common iliac a. & v.
Internal iliac a. & v.

External iliac a. & v.

Deep femoral a. & v.
Femoral a. & v.
Saphenous v.

Popliteal a. & v.

Anterior tibial a. & v.
Peroneal a.
Posterior tibial a. & v.

Dorsalis pedis a.
Dorsal venous arch

Key to abbreviations
a. Artery   **v.** Vein

The vascular system

All of the parts of the body are linked by the vascular system. This system is composed of three elements: the heart, blood vessels, and blood. There are three circulations involved: **cardiac** (through the heart), **pulmonary** (through the blood vessels in the lungs), and **systemic** (through the blood vessels in the rest of the body). Nutrients are delivered and waste products are removed from the body through the network of blood vessels in the body.

Vascular system circulations

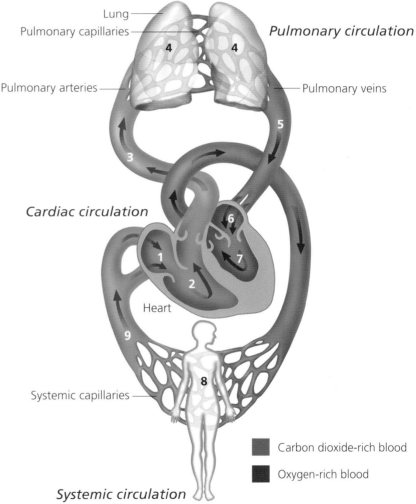

Lung
Pulmonary capillaries

Pulmonary circulation

Pulmonary arteries
Pulmonary veins

Cardiac circulation

Heart

Systemic capillaries

Carbon dioxide-rich blood
Oxygen-rich blood

Systemic circulation

1. Blood moves from the right atrium to the right ventricle by atrial contraction
2. Blood moves from the right ventricle to the pulmonary artery by ventricular contraction
3. Blood moves from the heart into the pulmonary arteries toward the lungs
4. **Blood moves into the capillaries in the lungs**
5. **Blood moves into the pulmonary veins back toward the heart**
6. Blood moves from the left atrium to the left ventricle by atrial contraction
7. Blood moves from the left ventricle into the aorta by ventricular contraction
8. **Blood moves into the capillaries in the body**
9. Blood returns to the heart through the venae cavae

The Vascular System

The heart

The heart is a four-chambered, muscular organ that functions as a powerful pump. About the size of a fist, the heart is located in the chest between the lungs, just to the left of center.

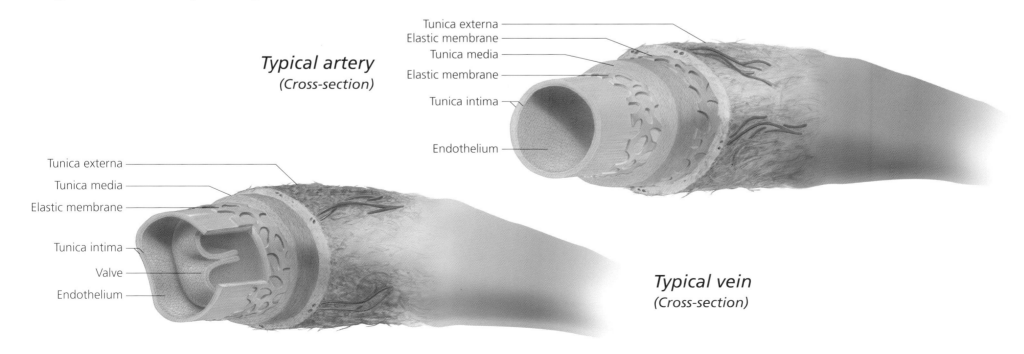

Heart
(Anterior view – partial cross-section)

Superior vena cava
Right pulmonary artery branches
Pulmonary trunk
Right pulmonary veins
Pulmonary semilunar valve
Right atrium
Tricuspid (right AV) valve
Chordae tendineae
Inferior vena cava
Right ventricle

Aorta
Left pulmonary artery
Left pulmonary veins
Left atrium
Aortic semilunar valve
Bicuspid (left AV) valve
Papillary muscle
Myocardium
Left ventricle
Interventricular septum
Trabeculae carneae

Heart
(Anterior view)

Left common carotid artery
Brachiocephalic artery
Superior vena cava
Ascending aorta
Right coronary artery
Right atrium
Right ventricle
Anterior cardiac vein
Right marginal artery
Small cardiac vein

Left subclavian artery
Aortic arch
Ligamentum arteriosum
Left pulmonary artery
Pulmonary trunk
Left auricle
Circumflex artery
Great cardiac vein
Anterior descending (interventricular) artery
Left ventricle
Apex

The blood vessels of the vascular system include three types: arteries, capillaries, and veins. Arteries carry blood away from the heart. The arteries branch into smaller vessels called **arterioles**, eventually branching to form a network of microscopic-sized capillaries. Every cell in the body is close to at least one capillary. After circulating through tissues, the capillaries merge to form small veins called **venules**. The venules merge to form veins, finally returning to the heart.

Typical artery
(Cross-section)

Tunica externa
Elastic membrane
Tunica media
Elastic membrane
Tunica intima
Endothelium

Typical vein
(Cross-section)

Tunica externa
Tunica media
Elastic membrane
Tunica intima
Valve
Endothelium

The Lymphatic System

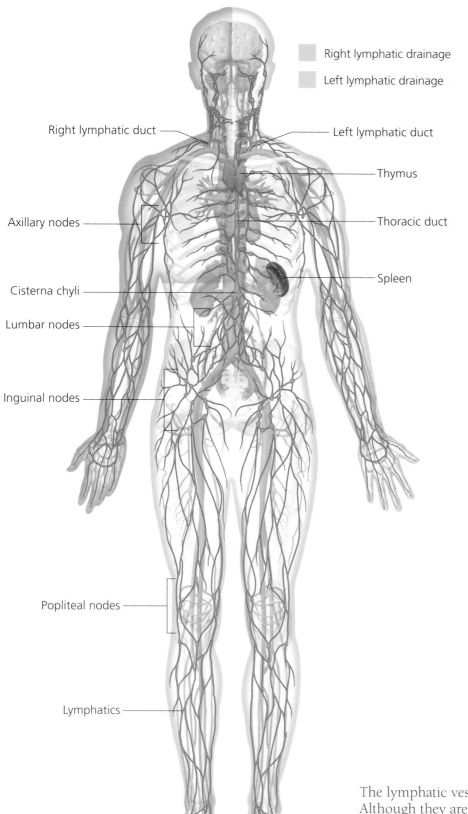

Right lymphatic drainage

Left lymphatic drainage

Right lymphatic duct

Left lymphatic duct

Thymus

Axillary nodes

Thoracic duct

Spleen

Cisterna chyli

Lumbar nodes

Inguinal nodes

Popliteal nodes

Lymphatics

The lymphatic system

The lymphatic system is an extensive network of vessels and nodes that forms a central part of the body's defenses against illness and injury. Foreign materials such as bacteria or dead cells are collected and transported through the lymph vessels, where they are filtered by the lymph nodes. The lymph vessels also drain excess fluid from the body's tissues, forming a fluid called **lymph**, and carry substances such as cholesterol and fat-soluble vitamins from the gastrointestinal system to the bloodstream.

All lymph passing through the lymphatic system is filtered by the lymph nodes lining the vessels. The lymph eventually flows into large channels called the thoracic and right lymphatic ducts and drains back into the bloodstream through the subclavian veins.

Lymph node

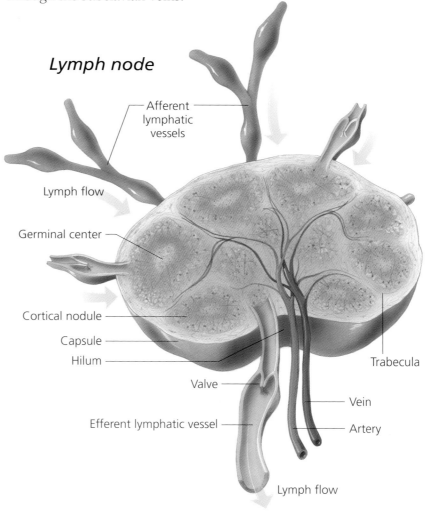

Afferent lymphatic vessels

Lymph flow

Germinal center

Cortical nodule

Capsule

Hilum

Valve

Vein

Artery

Trabecula

Efferent lymphatic vessel

Lymph flow

The lymphatic vessels are lined with hundreds of tiny bean-shaped organs called **lymph nodes**. Although they are scattered throughout the body, large clusters of lymph nodes are concentrated near specific areas such as the mammary glands and groin. Lymph nodes act as a barrier to infection by scavenging bacteria and other foreign materials from the lymph collected from the organs and tissues before it is returned to the bloodstream.

The Respiratory System

The respiratory system

Cells of the body get energy through aerobic metabolism, a process that uses oxygen and produces carbon dioxide as a waste product. The respiratory system provides the means to exchange these gases at the cellular level. The system includes the nose and nasal passages, the pharynx, larynx and trachea, the bronchi, and the lungs.

Respiratory mucosa

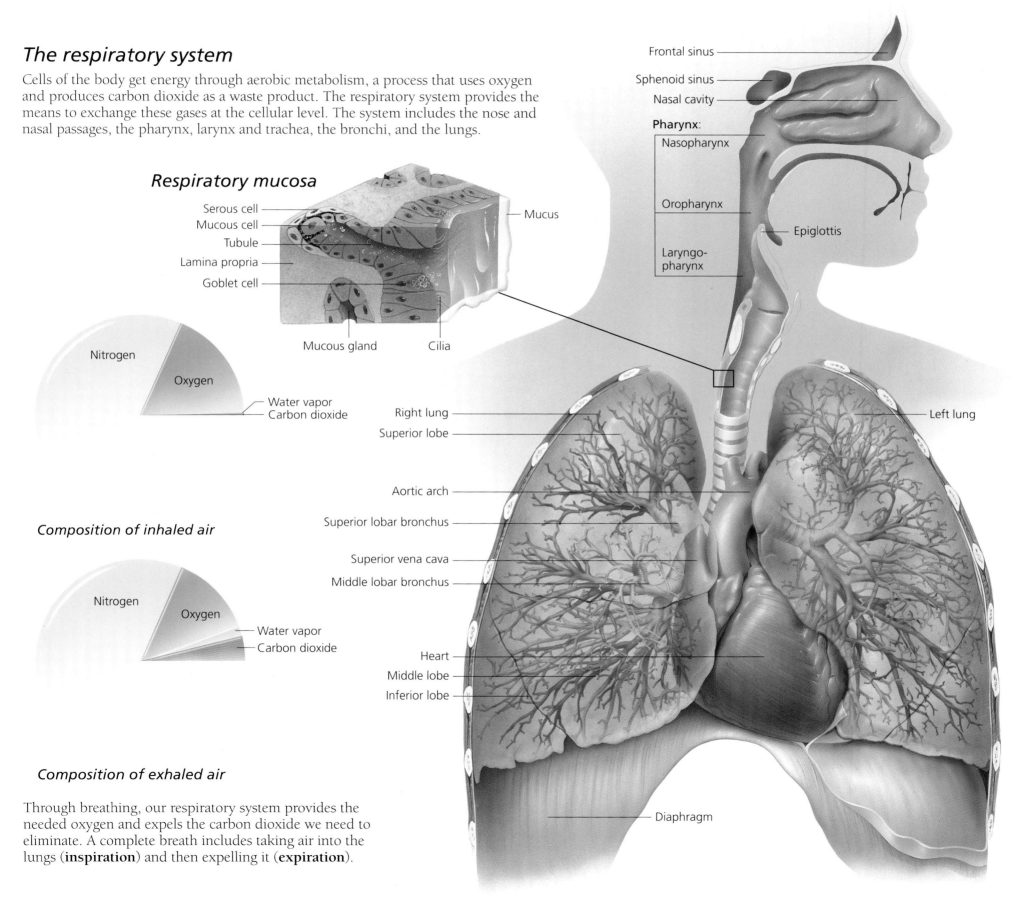

Serous cell
Mucous cell
Tubule
Lamina propria
Goblet cell
Mucus
Mucous gland
Cilia

Frontal sinus
Sphenoid sinus
Nasal cavity
Pharynx:
Nasopharynx
Oropharynx
Epiglottis
Laryngo-pharynx

Nitrogen
Oxygen
Water vapor
Carbon dioxide

Composition of inhaled air

Nitrogen
Oxygen
Water vapor
Carbon dioxide

Right lung
Superior lobe
Aortic arch
Superior lobar bronchus
Superior vena cava
Middle lobar bronchus
Heart
Middle lobe
Inferior lobe
Left lung
Diaphragm

Composition of exhaled air

Through breathing, our respiratory system provides the needed oxygen and expels the carbon dioxide we need to eliminate. A complete breath includes taking air into the lungs (**inspiration**) and then expelling it (**expiration**).

The Respiratory System

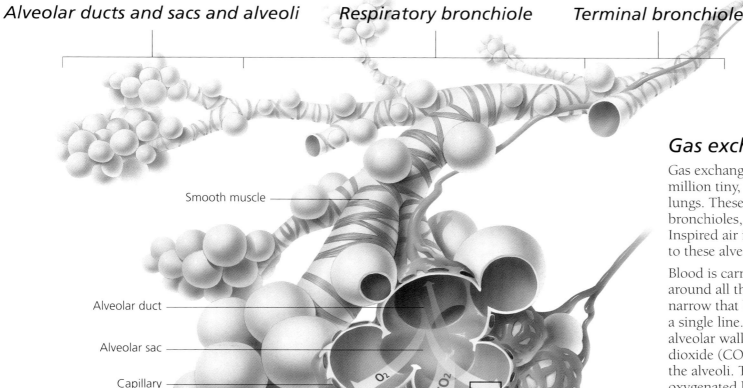

Alveolar ducts and sacs and alveoli   *Respiratory bronchiole*   *Terminal bronchiole*

Smooth muscle

Alveolar duct

Alveolar sac

Capillary

Alveolus

Gas exchange

Gas exchange occurs in the more than 600 million tiny, thin-membraned alveoli within the lungs. These alveoli reside along the respiratory bronchioles, alveolar ducts, and alveolar sacs. Inspired air is carried through the bronchioles to these alveoli.

Blood is carried to the capillaries that wrap around all the alveoli. These capillaries are so narrow that blood cells must pass through in a single line. Oxygen (O_2) diffuses across the alveolar wall into the blood cells as carbon dioxide (CO_2) diffuses from the blood into the alveoli. The CO_2 is exhaled. The newly oxygenated blood travels from the lungs to the heart to be circulated throughout the body.

Blood and gas circulation

One of the most critical jobs of the blood is transporting oxygen and carbon dioxide. During external respiration, oxygen diffuses from the air to the blood, where it bonds to hemoglobin. As blood passes through the tissues, the bond breaks, releasing oxygen. The lower the concentration of oxygen in the tissue, the more oxygen is released from the hemoglobin bond.

Carbon dioxide is carried away from the tissues by diffusing into red blood cells. CO_2 is dissolved in **plasma** (the water component of the blood) and reformed when the blood reaches the lungs, where it diffuses into the alveoli and is exhaled.

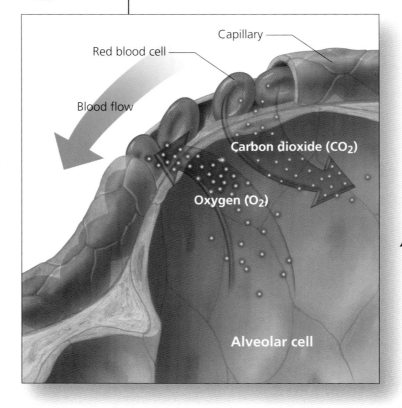

Capillary

Red blood cell

Blood flow

Carbon dioxide (CO_2)

Oxygen (O_2)

Alveolar cell

Alveolus and capillary

The Digestive System

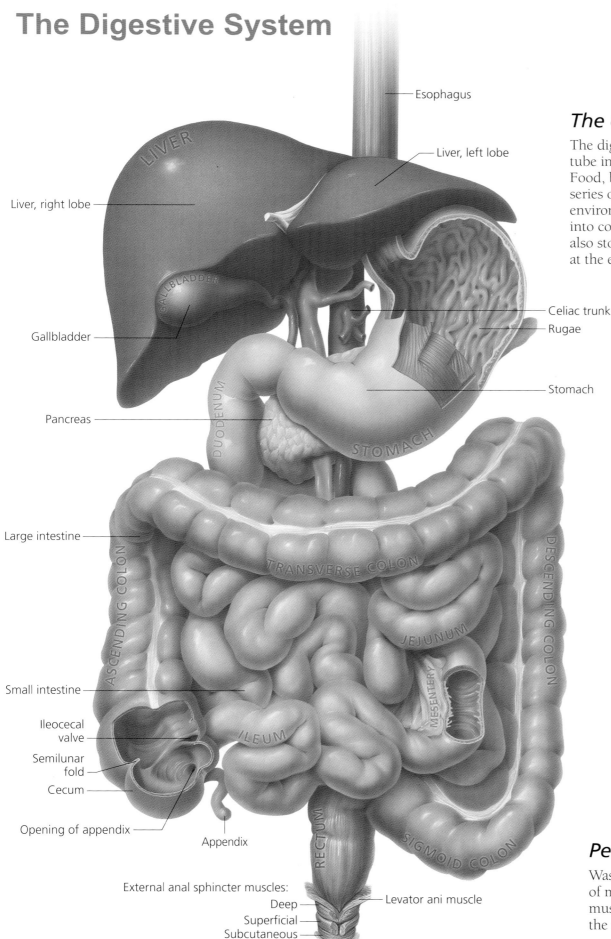

Esophagus

Liver, left lobe

LIVER

Liver, right lobe

GALLBLADDER

Gallbladder

Celiac trunk

Rugae

Stomach

Pancreas

DUODENUM

STOMACH

Large intestine

ASCENDING COLON

TRANSVERSE COLON

DESCENDING COLON

JEJUNUM

MESENTERY

Small intestine

Ileocecal valve

ILEUM

Semilunar fold

Cecum

Opening of appendix

Appendix

RECTUM

SIGMOID COLON

External anal sphincter muscles:

Deep

Levator ani muscle

Superficial

Subcutaneous

The digestive system

The digestive system, or gastrointestinal tract, is essentially a muscular tube in which intake, digestion, and absorption of nutrients take place. Food, broken down mechanically in the mouth, is propelled through a series of different secretory and absorptive environments. Within these environments, food is digested (broken down) by digestive enzymes into components small enough to be absorbed. The digestive system also stores unabsorbed components until they are ready to be expelled at the end of the gastrointestinal tract.

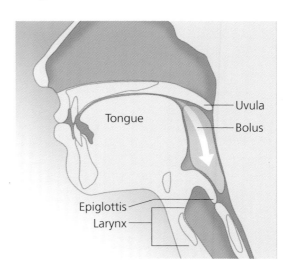

Uvula

Tongue

Bolus

Epiglottis

Larynx

Swallowing

The initial phase of the complex process of swallowing is voluntary. Once initiated, the remainder of the process is involuntary. Chewing mixes the food with saliva to form a **bolus**. As the bolus leaves the pharynx, the epiglottis, a flap-like valve, and the vocal cords close, blocking the trachea. Peristaltic action moves the bolus through the esophagus to the stomach.

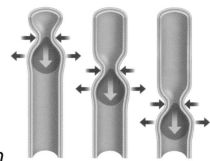

Peristaltic action

Waste material is moved through the digestive system by a series of muscle contractions called **peristalsis**. The contraction of the muscle behind the material moves it into the next section, where the muscle has relaxed.

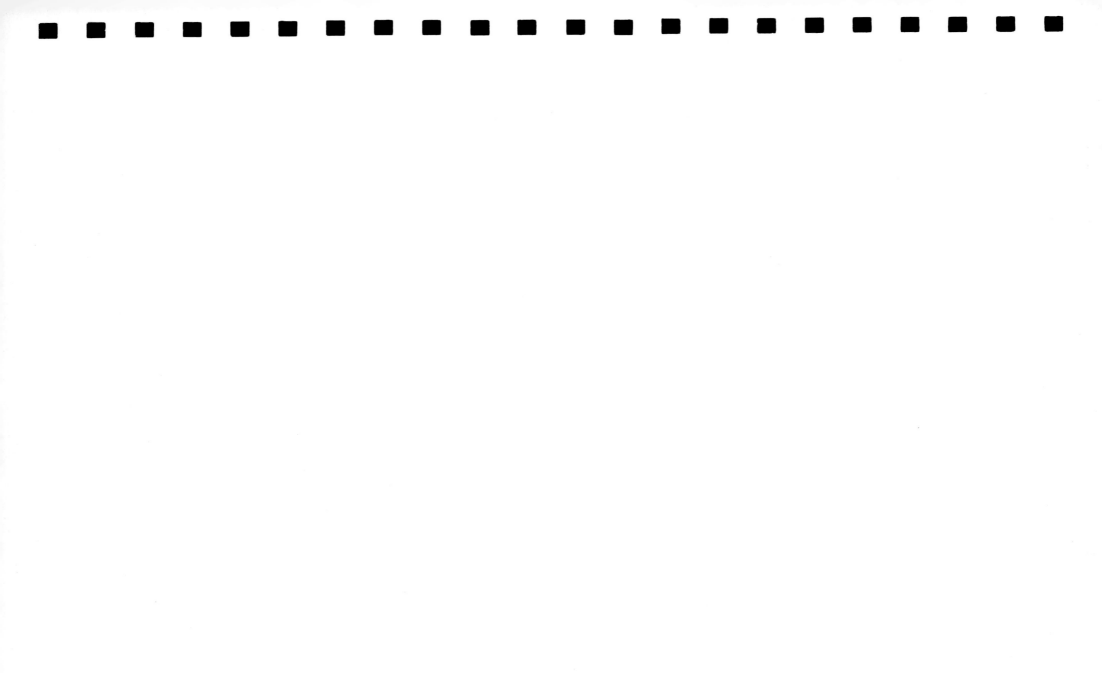

The Digestive System

Esophagus

The stomach

Swallowed food reaches the stomach after being pushed through the esophagus by wavelike muscular contractions called **peristalsis**. Once in the stomach, food mixes with hydrochloric acid and enzymes produced by the stomach lining to begin the digestion of proteins. This lining produces a layer of mucus to protect itself from the acid. The stomach also functions to store partially digested food (chyme) for processing later by the small intestine.

Rugae

Muscularis:
- Oblique
- Circular
- Longitudinal

Stomach

The small intestine

The small intestine consists of three areas, the duodenum, jejunum, and ileum. Digestion occurs throughout the entire length of the small intestine, accompanied by the absorption of the resulting molecules by the intestinal wall. **Villi**, projections of the lining of the small intestine, greatly increase the surface area of the absorptive membrane called the **epithelium**. Each cell of the epithelium has microvilli, which further increase this absorptive surface area.

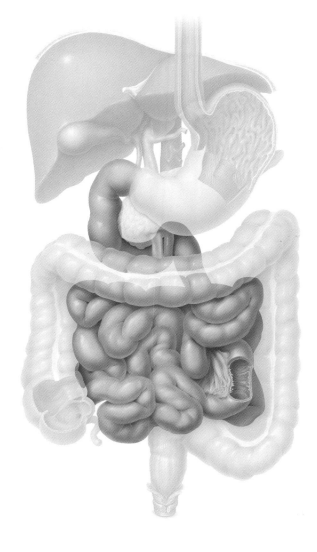

The large intestine

The large intestine consists of the cecum, the colon (ascending, transverse, descending, and sigmoid), and the rectum. As undigested material enters the large intestine, water and electrolytes are absorbed. The remaining waste is stored, formed, and expelled.

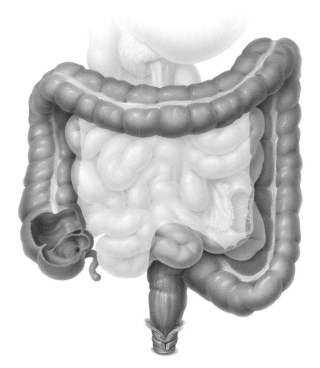

The Urinary System

The urinary system

The urinary system is responsible for three major functions in the body: removing wastes, maintaining normal water volume, and controlling acid-base balance in the bloodstream.

Urine formation begins within tiny functional units of the kidneys called **nephrons**. A complex three-step process of filtration, reabsorption, and secretion removes metabolic wastes, allows important substances such as glucose and water to be passed back into the blood, and eliminates toxins such as drugs and ammonia. The filtrate that results from this process is eventually diluted with water to produce **urine**.

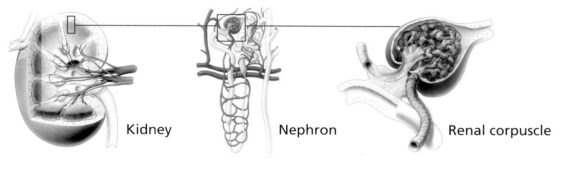

Kidney   Nephron   Renal corpuscle

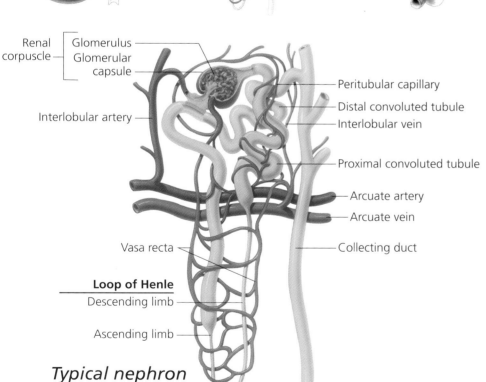

Renal corpuscle { Glomerulus / Glomerular capsule }

Interlobular artery

Peritubular capillary
Distal convoluted tubule
Interlobular vein
Proximal convoluted tubule
Arcuate artery
Arcuate vein
Collecting duct

Vasa recta

Loop of Henle
Descending limb
Ascending limb

Typical nephron

Each kidney contains more than a million nephrons, the microscopic units located in the outer renal cortex. A single nephron is made up of four components: the renal corpuscle, the proximal convoluted tubule, the loop of Henle, and the distal convoluted tubule. Nephrons regulate levels of water and soluble substances in the body by filtering the blood, reabsorbing water, glucose, and valuable ions such as potassium and sodium, and excreting excess water and waste products.

Kidney
Renal artery
Renal vein

Inferior vena cava
Abdominal aorta

Ureter

Bladder

The kidneys

The kidneys are located on each side of the spine at the back of the abdominal cavity. Each kidney is approximately four to five inches long and connects to the bladder via a narrow muscular tube called a **ureter**. We are normally born with a pair of kidneys, however we can survive with a single kidney.

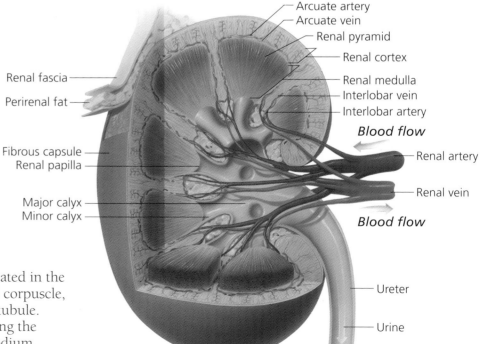

Arcuate artery
Arcuate vein
Renal pyramid
Renal cortex
Renal medulla
Interlobar vein
Interlobar artery

Blood flow

Renal fascia
Perirenal fat

Fibrous capsule
Renal papilla

Major calyx
Minor calyx

Renal artery

Renal vein

Blood flow

Ureter

Urine

The Reproductive System

Human reproduction

Humans reproduce by sexual reproduction involving male and female reproductive cells called **gametes**. The reproductive system includes:

- Reproductive organs called **gonads** that produce gametes and hormones
- Reproductive tracts for reception, storage, and transportation of gametes
- Accessory organs and glands for fluid secretion
- External genitalia

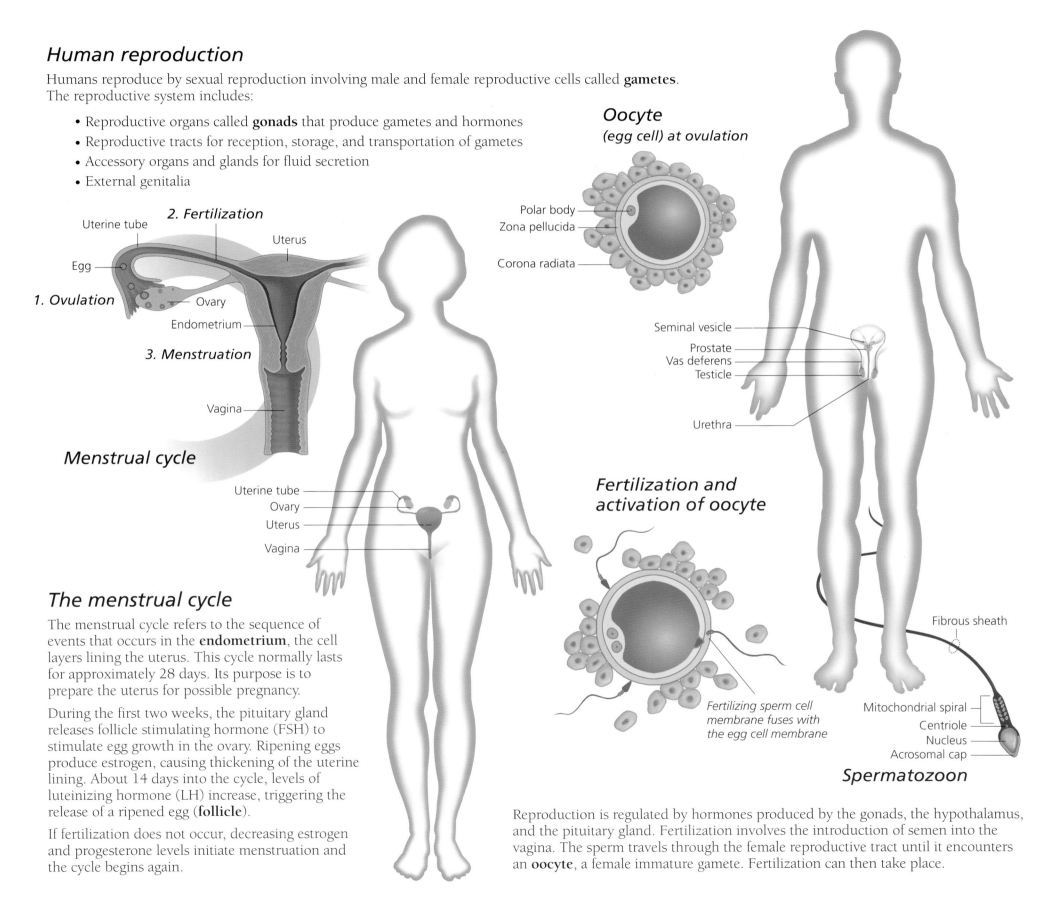

2. Fertilization

Uterine tube

Uterus

Egg

1. Ovulation

Ovary

Endometrium

3. Menstruation

Vagina

Menstrual cycle

Uterine tube
Ovary
Uterus
Vagina

Oocyte
(egg cell) at ovulation

Polar body
Zona pellucida

Corona radiata

Seminal vesicle
Prostate
Vas deferens
Testicle

Urethra

Fertilization and activation of oocyte

Fertilizing sperm cell membrane fuses with the egg cell membrane

Fibrous sheath

Mitochondrial spiral
Centriole
Nucleus
Acrosomal cap

Spermatozoon

The menstrual cycle

The menstrual cycle refers to the sequence of events that occurs in the **endometrium**, the cell layers lining the uterus. This cycle normally lasts for approximately 28 days. Its purpose is to prepare the uterus for possible pregnancy.

During the first two weeks, the pituitary gland releases follicle stimulating hormone (FSH) to stimulate egg growth in the ovary. Ripening eggs produce estrogen, causing thickening of the uterine lining. About 14 days into the cycle, levels of luteinizing hormone (LH) increase, triggering the release of a ripened egg (**follicle**).

If fertilization does not occur, decreasing estrogen and progesterone levels initiate menstruation and the cycle begins again.

Reproduction is regulated by hormones produced by the gonads, the hypothalamus, and the pituitary gland. Fertilization involves the introduction of semen into the vagina. The sperm travels through the female reproductive tract until it encounters an **oocyte**, a female immature gamete. Fertilization can then take place.